D0676242

Careers in
NURSING

your questions and answers

SECOND EDITION

WITHDRAWN FROM HAVERING COLLEGES
SIXTH FORM LIBRARY

HAVERING SIXTH FORM
COLLEGE LIBRARY

TROTMAN

This second edition published in 2000 in Great Britain
by Trotman and Company Limited,
2 The Green, Richmond, Surrey TW9 1PL
First edition by Joan Llewelyn Owens published in 1996

© Trotman and Company Limited 2000

British Library Cataloguing in Publication Data
A catalogue record for this book is available from the British Library
ISBN 0 85660 564 6

All rights reserved. No part of this publication may be
reproduced, stored in a retrieval system or transmitted in
any form or by any means, electronic and mechanical,
photocopying, recording or otherwise without prior permission
of Trotman and Company Limited.

Printed and bound in Great Britain
by Creative Print & Design (Wales) Ltd

Contents

Acknowledgements

The publishers would like to thank NHS Careers for providing recent details about work and training in the NHS. Further information can be obtained from NHS Careers, see page 40 for contact details.

What about working in nursing?

What do nurses do?

The role of nurses, according to the International Code for Nursing, is to promote health, to preserve life, to prevent illness and alleviate suffering. They fulfil this demanding role in a wide variety of environments, throughout the UK – and across the world – working closely with other health professionals as well as their patients.

Nurses are key members of the patient's healthcare team. That means they work alongside doctors, physiotherapists, and many others. They not only provide care but are involved in the planning of that care. This gives them an opportunity to influence the service given to patients.

Nurses are educators as well as carers. They help patients to understand the condition from which they are suffering and explain the aims of treatment. Nurses also advise and teach patients how to ward off illness and maintain good health. Nurses have a teaching role with parents too. If a sick child is better off treated at home rather than in hospital, nursing skills must be taught to the parents or guardians. In mental health nursing, counselling is an important part of a nurse's work.

In hospitals a named nurse may have specific responsibility for an individual patient, so that a rapport is built up. This occurs in the community, too, where a named district/community nurse is attached to one or more GP practices, although not directly employed by the GP. A midwife responsible for a particular mother-to-be will usually be at the labour and delivery of the baby, even if it is outside her working hours.

Working practices and the equipment used vary with the branch of nursing. For example, in a surgical ward, nurses will need to become competent in removing stitches and dressing wounds. Administration of medicines, giving injections and taking blood pressure are all examples of aspects of nursing.

Each patient's care plan identifies the needs of the patient, but as a nurse you will still have to think about what you are going to do. You will observe the patient closely, note how he or she is responding to treatment, discuss progress with others in the healthcare team, and if necessary alter your strategy.

With advances in technology and medical skills, and a shift towards primary healthcare, patients tend to be in hospital for shorter periods than in the past. Therefore, before a patient is discharged, nurses will be involved in discussions with other professionals and family members to ensure that the patient is adequately cared for once back at home.

In a hospital, nurses also have access to all kinds of sophisticated medical technology, which means that their level of knowledge is constantly advancing. In coronary care, they must be able to understand electrocardiographs and recognise the different traces of the heart so that if anything goes wrong they can inform the doctor. Nurses who work in intensive care units (ITUs), first go on a course which trains them on, for example, how to handle syringe drivers which administer pain-killers, ventilators and equipment for intravenous infusion.

The same facilities are not available in district nursing, when a nurse sees patients in their own homes. Nurses working in the community will have to plan their visits very carefully, take all they need with them, and maybe improvise on arrival.

What kind of people are nurses?

Nursing is a diverse and demanding job, attracting a range of dedicated and hard-working people. Nursing is open to both men and women, and although women still predominate, the proportion of men in the intake of students rises every year. Nurses, together with their health visitor and midwife colleagues, are the largest professional group in the National Health Service. Increasing numbers are also working in the private sector.

Nurses are well educated (to diploma in higher education or degree level) and highly skilled. They may be making life-and-death decisions so they have to have the knowledge, skills and experience to handle such responsibility.

They can be any age too. Although the minimum age to start a nursing career is $17\frac{1}{2}$, the NHS (the biggest employer) is keen to attract older applicants and to retrain career returners. Because nursing skills are always needed, and many of the techniques remain unchanged, it is always possible to have a career break, for instance to raise a family, and return to nursing later on.

What's the difference between registered nurse, health visitor and midwife?

Midwifery and health visiting are distinct professions from nursing, although some of the training is the same. Midwives provide support for the mother and her partner both before and after their baby's birth, assist in the delivery, and keep an eye on newborn babies and their families for several weeks. Midwives therefore work in the community and hospitals as well. They are the first link for new mothers to the maternity team, which includes doctors, nurses, physiotherapists and paediatricians.

When the family seems to be doing well, midwives hand over to the health visitors, who continue to keep in touch with the parents and monitor growth and development of the child.

Health visitors deal not only with babies, children and their parents, but with others as well. For example, they might act as counsellor to a family suffering bereavement, or offering support to someone trying to give up smoking.

It is useful to know which area you are interested in before you start your training, but there are opportunities to specialise later. Health visitors normally train as registered nurses first and then study for a post-registration qualification, but there are some degree courses offering students dual qualification as registered nurses and as health visitors. There are both direct entry and post-registration midwifery programmes, too (see page 36).

What sorts of jobs are there?

The quick answer is – a tremendous variety. The main types of career are in the four branches of nursing (adult, mental health, child and learning disabilities), or midwifery or health visiting. Nurses work with other professionals in a range of different environments – such as GP practices, schools and in the community. Here's a brief outline of the ways you could specialise and where you might work.

The four branches of nursing

Adult branch

In this branch students learn how to provide appropriate care for people with chronic and acute physical illness, in hospital, in health centres and GP surgeries, and in the community. Hospital stays are generally much shorter than in the past, and some surgical procedures are conducted on a day basis (eg in an outpatients clinic). Within the adult branch, there is scope to specialise in, for instance, orthopaedics, accident and emergency, cardiac care, intensive care or care of the elderly. Nurses can also become theatre nurses, assisting the surgeon during operations. District and practice nursing are discussed on pages 8–9.

Mental health branch

There are considerable differences between nursing people with physical illnesses or injuries and those with mental illnesses. One misconception is that this type of nursing involves dealing with violent behaviour. This doesn't often occur. Together with other members of the team (such as GPs, psychiatrists and social workers), mental health nurses try to discover what has caused the problem in the first place and help to plan the care and treatment.

Mental illness is not uncommon, and can be a severe case of depression, stress or anxiety, which needs professional help. Every person is treated as an individual, and treatment is tailored to individual needs. People are mainly treated in the community, in their own homes and at local health centres, although some may need hospitalisation from time to time.

In mental health work, you will see patients over longer periods of time than the nurse in the adult branch. As a result you have greater opportunities to develop relationships with your patients and use those relationships for their benefit. Importantly, you will be helping both patients and their families to deal with any stigma they feel is attached to the illness, and giving them confidence, and helping them to understand the treatment.

Child branch

Nursing a sick child is not the same as nursing a miniature adult. Children can become ill very quickly, and they can recover quickly, too. A child could be a newborn baby in intensive care, or a 13-year-old with a broken arm. Nurses have to be intuitive – ie able to interpret a child's behaviour, as the child might not be able to explain what is wrong. They need to know how children develop, and how illness can interfere with their growth and learning.

Nursing children often means working closely with families. You may need to teach a parent how to look after the patient, as it is so much less frightening for the child to have a familiar person involved in the care, and when possible the child is nursed at home. Parents are also likely to be worried and distressed by the injury or ill health their child suffers, so you need to be calm, reassuring and sensitive towards them and the whole family too.

Learning disabilities branch

Some people with severe learning disabilities often have physical and mental disabilities as well. In addition to their special needs, they require the same sort of healthcare as other adults and children. The main aspect of the work is to help people to improve their lifestyles and to participate in society. It might mean teaching certain basic skills, like washing and dressing, or interactive ones, like using money and travel by public transport.

Most people with learning disabilities live in the community, some with their families, some in special homes, while some are able to live on their own. Progress with such patients can be very slow, so as a nurse in this field you will need exceptional patience and commitment. You also need to be sensitive and a very good communicator – able to listen as well as make yourself understood. Certainly you need to become very close to those you care for, and work well with other carers, such as psychologists, therapists and special teachers.

Midwifery

The midwife's role isn't just in the delivery of babies – it can start as early as pre-conceptual care, advising the prospective mother how to get her body into the ideal condition to conceive. Midwives practise both in hospital and the community, giving antenatal (before birth) care, delivering babies and supporting both the mother and her partner, before, during and after the birth. They are part of a team and cooperate closely with obstetricians, GPs and health visitors.

Health visiting

Health visitors work not just with mothers and babies – their task is to promote good health and to prevent ill health in the community as a whole. They talk to prospective mothers about preparation for child-birth, and when a new baby is a few weeks old, they usually take over from the midwife to visit the family and discuss the baby's progress. They regularly call on families with children up to five years old, and in the home they advise both adolescents and adults on a variety of matters, including the problems of old age. When someone is discharged from hospital, they can do a great deal to help families continue to care for the patient at home.

District nursing

District nurses work in teams of qualified and unqualified staff, headed by someone who is the hospital equivalent of a ward sister. They cooperate with many other agencies, including the health and social services. Most district nurses are attached to one or more general practices, although employed by the local National Health Trust.

The district nurse's patients tend to be seen at home, throughout the community. Particularly in rural areas, some district nurses have a double or a triple role, being qualified in district nursing, health visiting and midwifery.

Many nursing procedures can be carried out in a patient's home rather than in hospital. District nurses attend people with illnesses like pneumonia; those who are having high-tech care such as kidney dialysis, gastric feeding or chemotherapy; and people who have terminal illnesses and prefer to be in their own homes with their families for the end of their lives.

They have a monitoring role when people are chronically sick and particularly frail, watching over people with wounds and leg ulcers, problems with incontinence and general disabilities. They also have a health promotion role, talking to groups of people who might be at risk: for instance, about the prevention of hypothermia for the elderly.

Practice nursing

Practice nurses are based at the doctor's surgery, health centre or specialist clinic, where they have a variety of duties. In a general clinic, they check blood pressure, take blood samples for analysis, give immunisation treatments, apply dressings and remove stitches. Other procedures that might be the responsibility of the practice nurse, either in the surgery or at a specialist clinic, would be to monitor and look after 'well babies', 'well women', diabetics, asthmatics; to give family planning advice; and, for example, to inform people going abroad about health risks in different parts of the world, and give the necessary jabs. Practice nurses may also be responsible for ordering medical equipment and other stores and cleaning any instruments that have been used.

Occupational nursing

Either as individual practitioners or as part of a team, occupational health nurses work together with management and employees to reduce sickness and cut absence rates in workplaces. The key elements of occupational nursing are the prevention of ill health; the promotion of health and safety; the provision of care for people who become sick or injured at work; the monitoring of the environment; and managing an occupational health service to meet the specific needs of the organisation by which they are employed.

School nursing

The school nurse has a vital role in encouraging children to adopt healthy lifestyles. School nurses give information, support and advice to individual children and their parents, and offer support to teachers in providing health education within the national curriculum. It used to be the case that each child reaching school age underwent a school entry medical conducted by the school doctor, assisted by the school nurse. The nurse also carried out vision and hearing screening. Now most primary health teams have taken on the role of pre-school child health surveillance. This is usually undertaken by health visitors with the general practitioner. The school nurse usually conducts healthcare interviews, which involve not only the screening of vision, hearing, height and weight, but a holistic assessment of the health needs of the child and his or her family.

On the health promotion side, the school nurse may give one-to-one teaching and counselling or plan and deliver group health education sessions. The nurse administers certain medicines, attends to minor ailments and carries out first aid. School nurses may also instruct staff in first aid.

What qualifications will I need?

To practice as a nurse you need to be qualified as a registered nurse (RN). All registered nurses and midwives take either a diploma or degree 'pre-registration' course (see page 35).

The minimum age of entry to nurse training is 17½ (17 in Scotland). For the diploma course you will normally need at least five GCSE passes or equivalent at grade C or above. These must include English and preferably maths; a science subject is also useful and might be required on some courses (especially for midwifery). Some vocational qualifications, such GNVQ Advanced Level or NVQ Level 3, are acceptable. (You may be able to get a healthcare assistant role in a hospital, where you can train to NVQ levels 2 and 3. If you are working for the NHS, you may have access to employment schemes where you can retain your salary while taking the nurse training programme.)

Different schools of nursing will have their own requirements and it is worthwhile ringing to check, and getting hold of prospectuses to see what the course covers. Mature students may be offered the opportunity to sit the UKCC (UK Central Council for Nursing, Midwifery and Health Visiting) written entry test, known as the 'DC test'.

For degree programmes you will require at least two A-levels or equivalent, in addition to passes at GCSE. Each institution will give details of individual requirements in its prospectus. For example, you might be required to have a science subject at A-level, and have achieved certain grades.

What personal skills and attitudes are needed?

First and foremost a nurse must want to look after others. The ability to make people comfortable will come with training. It is a combination of technical skills (for no one will be comfortable if a nurse is not competent) and human skills – ie the ability to work with all types of people and adapt to their needs.

Admissions tutors also look for maturity, confidence, communication skills and motivation. You will be part of a multidisciplinary team, including doctors, physiotherapists, anaesthetists and many others, so being able to work as a member of a team is important. Good powers of observation can save lives; so can quick thinking. Nurses need a calm and balanced personality, which means that they are capable of working in emergency conditions, and under stress.

When working with children and people with learning disabilities, it is important to be able to interpret reactions, for often they will not be able to tell you what is wrong. Children's nurses also require tremendous sensitivity and imagination.

Nurses should have good time-management skills coupled with flexibility. District nurses, for example, must plan their visiting schedules carefully to make best use of their time, but be ready to improvise when things don't go according to plan. In accident and emergency, you will need the ability to prioritise and to make swift decisions as to what is most important. This should come with training and experience.

In mental health nursing, you will need the ability to form therapeutic relationships with patients and their families. Much of the behaviour of people who are mentally ill may appear bizarre, but nurses must be non-judgemental. While patience is necessary at all times, it is one of the most essential qualities for someone working with people with learning disabilities; progress can be very slow, with many setbacks.

All nurses must enjoy responsibility, and as they progress in their career and take charge of junior staff, they need the leadership skills to motivate a team. Management skills are essential to make career progress into ward management or general hospital management.

How competitive an area is it?

This in an area in which is it reasonably easy to obtain work – if you have the qualifications and the qualities that make a good nurse. However, it is a very responsible job and the only way of getting a position is by becoming a student nurse and taking a pre-registration course – either a diploma in higher education or a degree in nursing.

Some of the courses do fill up quickly, so get your application in as soon as you can. The application period is from September to the end of June for courses beginning at the earliest in the autumn of the following year. Applications for diploma courses are through the Nursing and Midwives Admissions Service (NMAS) and for degree courses through the Universities and Colleges Admissions Service (UCAS) (see pages 41—42). In July, August and September you can apply directly to the university of your choice.

NHS Careers is a good place to start for applications advice. Also, get hold of prospectuses, and make a visit to colleges that interest you. There will be competition for pre-registration courses, so make sure you have the right qualifications, work experience and personal attributes to win a place.

What are the good and bad aspects of the work?

No one pretends that nursing is an easy option – 24-hour cover must be maintained, and having to work shifts can play havoc with a nurse's personal life. Nursing is physically tiring and sometimes emotionally draining. It is no easy task to deal with a worried parent of a very sick baby, and it is even more stressful when patients die.

But the rewards can be tremendous. In all branches of nursing there are upbeat moments, such as when a dangerously ill child makes a dramatic recovery, or nurses realise they have saved lives by detecting life-threatening conditions. Even when nursing the terminally ill, to enable someone to have a pain-free, dignified death, surrounded by family, it is certainly worthwhile.

As a registered nurse you will be bound by a code of professional conduct that includes ethical and moral issues, and guidance given by the UK Central Council for Nursing, Midwifery and Health Visiting (UKCC). Nurses register with the UKCC every three years after demonstrating professional practice development. When you are dealing with people's lives and their health, inevitably there will be difficult ethical decisions to be taken. For instance, you as well as the doctors may be involved in a decision as to whether life support should be withdrawn, or what to do in the case of someone critically ill refusing treatment. You will need tact to deal with patients and their families, and be prepared sometimes to be the bearer of bad news.

Nurses do not just deal with people who are unwell or injured. School nurses, for example, help to educate young people and are sensitive to the diseases likely to affect them. Midwives enjoy working in the community as well as in hospital and get to know expectant mothers during the months before birth. Helping to bring a healthy baby into the world is extremely rewarding, and so is helping new parents learn to feed and care for their newborn child. Practice nurses have huge variety in their work, and help many different types of people with treatment and advice on a range of healthcare issues. Those working with people with learning disabilities can teach important skills and therefore give self-confidence.

In all forms of nursing one of the main aims is to help people who need support to become independent again, so every case brings challenges and rewards. The tremendous variety of a nursing career and all the new developments that improve the quality of care are fulfilling for many nurses. Every day is different, so it is impossible to be bored.

What sort of expectations do you have? Surveys of student nurses have shown that many anticipate these positive aspects of a nursing career:

- having responsibility
- having job satisfaction
- working in a friendly atmosphere
- using skills fully
- being able to use initiative.

These are all true, and you will gain additional skills as you learn to bring your own training and aptitudes to a multidisciplinary team. On the downside, many trainee nurses did not expect flexible or part-time working and good pay. This is not necessarily the case. While it is true that the majority of nurses feel they are poorly paid compared with other professional groups, part-time work and flexible arrangements to suit those with family responsibilities is today more likely in a nursing career than many others. And for ambitious and experienced nurses, there are opportunities to progress to well-paid and responsible jobs in management, or as a clinical nurse specialist, becoming an expert in your chosen field.

If you are interested in this line of work, you probably realise that caring for people brings many rewards. Nurses feel they are privileged in the close relationship they often have with patients. In giving healthcare they are assisting people to reach their maximum potential. They are also finding many new and interesting opportunities opening up, as they take over some of the roles previously reserved for doctors.

Where will I work?

Nurses work in hospitals (both NHS and private), hospices, health centres, GP surgeries and in the community. They are based throughout the country, in cities, towns and rural areas. Large hospitals have a tremendous variety of departments or specialisms; for example, general medical and surgical wards, children's wards, and special interest areas such as orthopaedics, gynaecology and obstetrics, cardiac care, intensive care, the operating theatre, ear nose and throat (ENT), outpatients, accident and emergency, and care of the elderly. There are some specialist hospitals, too, dealing with such areas as eyes, neurological problems and mental health.

Based in the community, practice nurses see patients who visit health and medical centres. Health visitors may also operate from these centres, providing a service to the population of a GP, or working in a certain geographical area, making frequent visits to patients' homes.

District nurses, who also visit patients, are usually attached to one or more general practice. The school nurse spends most of the day in schools, while the occupational nurse works in industry, commerce, hospitals, universities and colleges. Midwives are based in hospitals, where they conduct normal births in the delivery suite, and mother and baby clinics. They also visit women and families at home, for home births, to help educate them on childcare, and check on new babies.

Opportunities also occur for nurses to join the Armed Forces, to work for the Prison Service, and to work in addiction units.

Who will I work with?

As a nurse you will work alongside a wide range of healthcare professionals. Nurses are members both of a nursing team and of a wider multidisciplinary team, including GPs, hospital doctors, consultants, physiotherapists, occupational therapists, dietitians, and many others.

In a children's ward nurses also cooperate with teachers and play therapists, sometimes with nursery nurses. They work with the child's whole family, teaching them how to care for a sick child and administer injections and medicines.

In mental health other members of the professional team will include psychiatrists and psychologists. In the nursing of people with learning disabilities, nurses work alongside special teachers and social workers. They also work with relatives and carers.

What will I earn?

Your salary will depend on where you are based, your job, your level of experience and how many hours you work. London salaries will be slightly more than elsewhere, and if you work part-time, you will probably be paid on a pro rata basis (ie proportionally – if you work half the number of hours in a year, you get paid half the annual salary). As a student nurse on a diploma course you will get at least £4600 a year (see page 37). Once you qualify you will be on a graded salary scale, with your salary increasing as you gain more experience and responsibility. The following figures are recommended national rates of basic pay in 2000 for the nursing grades, not including London weighting.*

Grade A	£9,000–£11,010
Grade B	£10,660–£12,135
Grade C	£12,135–£14,890
Grade D	£14,890–£16,445
Grade E	£15,920–£19,220
Grade F	£17,655–£21,635
Grade G	£20,830–£24,090
Grade H	£23,270–£26,610
Grade I	£25,770–£29,205

Nurses and midwives also earn on average over 10% of their basic pay in allowances, eg for working night shifts and weekends. There are other types of career such as nurse consultants and those in health service management, who can earn over £40,000pa with the right qualifications, experience and seniority.

(*Source: NHS Careers, 'Pay Information' leaflet.)

What are the hours and holidays like?

Nursing care is provided 24 hours a day, seven days a week, and over bank holidays. Staffing levels vary at different times during the day and week. With the exception of specialist areas, such as intensive care units, the level of staffing in hospitals at night is lower than the average of day staffing.

The basic working week for nurses is 37½ hours, including shifts and, in most places, night duty. In hospitals shift systems take into account the differing staffing needs at different times of the day or the week (fewer staff may be needed at the weekend when there are fewer operating sessions). One common system involves a combination of staff working early and late shifts with a permanent night staff. Staff working a mix of early and late shifts will normally work weekends and public holidays. Night shifts on average are around 11 hours.

In the NHS, flexible and part-time work is available to suit different personal circumstances and commitments, but again this will depend on where you work and the team you work with. Agency work is one way of only working when you want to, but you don't get paid holidays.

If you work in a general practice or other clinic, there will be fairly standard working hours when the clinic is open. But you may be 'on call' at other times, ready to answer an emergency at night or weekends. Midwives, for instance, can't ensure expectant mothers give birth in normal working hours!

Qualified nurses in the NHS have five weeks' holiday (25 days) a year, plus bank holidays or days off in lieu.

Will I meet the public?

As a nurse, you will meet the public of all ages, from newly born babies to the very aged. The sort of people you meet will depend on the type of nursing you do. Their circumstances will differ widely. There will be the affluent, the reasonably well off and the very poor. In a children's ward or when visiting children at home, you will meet the parents and siblings as well. If you work with disabled people, you will meet their carers.

As a district nurse you could work with a range of people in a wide variety of places – for example, in a run-down city area you might have to visit the desperately ill living in appalling poverty, prisoners, prostitutes or drug addicts – all sorts of people who it may be hard to treat for many different reasons.

In occupational nursing, the nurse meets everyone from the worker on the shop floor or office to the managing director. The school nurse is responsible for the healthcare of teachers as well as pupils.

Are the prospects good for my career?

Your prospects are very good, as there is a shortage of nurses in most hospitals. It is estimated that the NHS needs to recruit approximately 20,000 qualified nurses each year simply to replace those who leave the service. Meanwhile the demand for nursing staff is increasing and will continue to do so.

Employment prospects do vary with the specialty. There are comparatively few employment difficulties for nurses qualifying in children's health or mental health. Practice nursing is a growth area. Over all, there is an extremely low level of unemployment among nurses, and it is unlikely that a qualified nurse looking for work would be unemployed for long. Even taking a career break, for instance to travel, raise a family or gain other qualifications, will not damage your prospects. You can always be retrained, and the maturity and life skills you gain outside the profession are considered a valuable addition to your qualifications. Once you are qualified as an RN, if you have dependants and want to work at only certain times, part-time or flexible work and job-share schemes might well be available to you.

Or maybe you are ambitious to move up the career ladder into more senior posts? That's possible too, depending on your talent and commitment. On qualification a student becomes a staff nurse, and opportunities occur for promotion to senior staff nurse, junior and senior sister (or charge nurse in the case of men), and to become a nurse manager. There is nothing to stop a nurse reaching the highest management posts in the NHS, working with medical and administration managers to oversee how healthcare is delivered in hospitals and trusts.

Opportunities occur, too, in advanced clinical specialisms, such as diabetes, plastics and burns, infection control, oncology and breast care. A nurse who specialises in a clinical area and also gets involved in research and teaching could eventually become a nurse consultant at a very high level. Nurse education is another big employment area – teaching both new nurses and giving specialist courses for qualified nurses who want to develop skills in a particular area.

Experienced registered nurses are also recruited by the nursing services of the Armed Forces – Queen Alexandra's Royal Naval Nursing Service (QARNNS), Queen Alexandra's Royal Army Nursing Corps (QARANC) and Princess Mary's Royal Air Force Nursing Service (PMRAFNS) .

What about training at work?

When you are studying for your diploma or degree, you will spend a considerable amount of time in hospitals and other healthcare environments to develop your practical skills, at the same time as you learn the theory. Effectively you are training as soon as you start to study.

As a qualified nurse, health visitor or midwife you will be expected to stay up to date with the latest developments in clinical and professional practice and to become a lifelong learner. That means you will be developing your skills even when qualified, and it is likely courses will be available to you if you want to specialise or need refresher training. Post-registration courses of varying length are available in many subjects, from accident and emergency to urology; there are courses on chemotherapy, coronary care, intensive care, liver disorders and transplantation, and many other fields.

You will be encouraged to undertake further training in line with your interests, abilities and aspirations with regard to your career. If you have qualified by means of a diploma, it will be possible to add further accredited units to convert your qualification into a full honours degree. Many nurses also study for postgraduate qualifications in their particular interest. Career returners to the NHS (for instance, after a gap to have children), are given the support and training needed to refresh their professional skills.

Will I need other languages for the work?

No, you won't need them, but they are always useful, especially if you hope to nurse overseas (see next section). If you work in a city with a large minority population of non-English speakers, knowing their language would mean you could communicate more easily, understand their needs and help them to understand treatment. Translators are often available to hospitals if needed.

Will I be able to work overseas or travel for my job?

There are numerous opportunities to travel abroad and work as a nurse. There is complete freedom of movement for registered nurses in Europe, as training in the UK meets the standards laid down in EU directives for general nursing. If you are intending to work abroad, you should first contact the appropriate licensing authority to find out the requirements for practising as a registered nurse in that country. Members of either the Royal College of Nursing or of the trade union Unison can obtain guidance from these organisations.

It is also possible to undertake a period of voluntary or missionary work overseas, with organisations like Voluntary Service Overseas (VSO), the Church Missionary Society and the Baptist Missionary Society.

If you take a commission as a nursing officer in one of the nursing services attached to the Armed Services, you are bound to do a certain amount of travelling to different parts of the country. It is usual to move from one type of appointment to another, to give you the widest possible experience in preparation for senior rank. However, overseas postings are not that common. When UK Forces are involved in theatres of war, medical and nursing personnel run field hospitals, hospital ships, and are members of mobile surgical teams.

What are the recent developments in this area?

Primary healthcare

Since the 1990 NHS and Community Care Act, one of the main changes has been the shift towards 'primary healthcare'. This is about ensuring that the population has healthcare provision within the community, at local health centres, nearer to home, and even at home.

People spend a shorter time in hospital, and sick children in particular go home as soon as possible. They are then cared for by their families with the support of a growing number of paediatric nurses based in the community. Nurses trained in the learning disabilities branch now work in a wider range of settings. Many of their clients now live at home or in supported settings. The same occurs in the case of the mentally ill, many of whom are cared for in the community.

Nursing responsibilities

Another change that is gradual, but has an impact on nurse training and responsibilities, is in the working relationships between healthcare professionals. Doctors and nurses are encouraged to work closely together and share their skills and experience, in order to deliver care more flexibly. For example, junior doctors and nurses might share tasks like phlebotomy (taking blood samples), cannulation (inserting needles into veins), assessing, investigating, treating and discharging patients, counselling and pain relief. Nurses with a particular clinical specialism and many years in the nursing profession might be responsible for overseeing some services that doctors used to run, such as pre-admission clinics, out-patient clinics, minor injury services and cardiology daycare.

There has also been a growth of nurse practitioners, specially qualified to work independently of doctors, though they will refer patients in need of medical treatment. Nurse prescribing has come about, too, to an extent. District nurses and health visitors at a number of sites throughout the country can prescribe some remedies and medicines for their patients. A health visitor, for instance, visiting a mother and new baby at home, may notice that the baby has oral thrush. Now she can write out a prescription for the appropriate remedy and explain how to use the medication as well as giving feeding advice. This saves the mother from having to take her baby to see the doctor, as she would have done in the past.

Training and education

Nurse education is currently undergoing review, too. From September 2000 a number of colleges and universities across the UK have introduced a new model of education. The main differences are to give trainees more options and greater flexibility through a credit system. Trainees could accrue credits on the course, which means they could take a break from studying, and return to it later, perhaps after employment in the NHS as a support worker. They will also be able to gain credits towards qualification for previous learning (whether in education or by experience). The Common Foundation Programme is reduced to one year, with two years specialising in one of the four nursing branches.

Meanwhile, once qualified, further training opportunities are open to nurses now – some nurses choose to qualify in alternative therapies, such as reflexology, to help relieve pain and stress among patients. (You don't have to be a registered nurse to train in alternative therapies, but you do have to follow training programmes to qualify and practise legally. For more information on alternative careers, see the booklist for suggestions on further reading.)

What impact has new technology had on this work?

The technology revolution has not had a massive impact on the type of patient care given by nurses, but it has on the administrative aspects of healthcare. Most patient information, in hospitals and at GPs' surgeries, is stored on computers and nurses use these systems to input data and access patients' histories. In many hospitals and community settings, care planning is also computerised.

There are some fields where technological advances have provided tools for use in treatment. For instance, computerised sensory stimulation and interactive learning systems are especially useful in helping people with learning disabilities. The theatre nurse might be involved in surgical procedures that use the latest technology, and in intensive care monitoring of patients' progress is usually done by sophisticated electronic equipment.

NHS Direct, established in 1998, is an example of information and communications technology (ICT) being used to improve the efficiency of healthcare provision. People can telephone to describe their symptoms to trained staff like nurses. Using both their nursing skills and computer programs to help identify the likely cause, staff are able to suggest courses of action, such as over-the-counter (non-prescription) remedies, contacting a GP or visiting an accident and emergency department at hospital. (There is some controversy about this service, and currently available statistics do not prove that it reduces the number of visits to doctors and hospitals.)

Could I become famous?

Unless you forsake nursing for show business, politics or journalism, it is unlikely that the general public will get to know your name. Claire Rayner, the agony aunt, trained as a nurse. So did Baroness Cox, and there are several other nurses in parliament. The actress Julie Walters is nursing trained, too.

Some nurses are widely known because of the prominence of the posts they hold. If you read nursing journals and follow healthcare issues on the news and in the national press, you will become familiar with the names of people who are active in the field. Within the medical world and sometimes within a wider sphere, certain nurses have a name because they follow up their special interests and become experts in a particular field. For example, between 1960 and 1986, Betty Parsons taught 20,000 women, including the Queen, to 'relax for pregnancy and for life'.

The most famous nurse of all, of course, was Florence Nightingale. It's worth knowing a bit about this influential person – she founded modern nursing and showed the world what a very important role it is.

Could I work independently?

Nurses are increasingly recognised as autonomous practitioners, often being the first to see patients and to undertake certain treatments. In such cases it is they who make the decision as to whether the patient needs to be referred to a medical practitioner. However, they always remain members of a multiskilled team, and they have to be able to work closely with that team.

So, you can't set up in business for yourself as a nurse, but for more independence you could join an agency and accept work when it fits in with your life. But you must be well qualified and flexible to ensure you get the work you want through an agency. You must also be a good team player and quick to learn in different environments. Most nurses and midwives who work in this way have had substantial experience already.

How can I find out more about the work?

It's a good idea to know as much as possible about the work before starting a pre-registration degree or diploma course. You should read all you can about nursing – look at books, magazines and read newspapers to keep up to date with changes in the health service. Your local careers office will have useful books to look at, and information is available from the Department of Health and NHS Careers (see page 40).

You might want to get involved in weekend voluntary work in a community or healthcare setting, if there's anything you can do locally. Check libraries and community centres for this type of work – for example St John Ambulance, or work with children or the elderly. See if a hospital near you will let you have a period of work experience, or take a Red Cross course.

Talk to anyone you know who works in nursing, or any other of the professions allied to medicine (eg physiotherapy, radiography, chiropody and occupational therapy). All people in nursing and medicine work as a team, so by talking to any members of that team you will find out more about what is involved in patient care. Ask them what they do, who they work with, what type of people they treat, what are the good and bad points of their work – and anything else you want to know about.

What should I do now to prepare?

- Make sure in the first place that you are studying hard for the right educational qualifications. Get prospectuses from universities and colleges running degree and diploma courses to check which GCSE subjects you need. These will also give you some idea of the scope of the course and subjects you will have to study on a nursing course.

- Do as much relevant background reading as possible, studying journals such as *Nursing Times* and *Nursing Standard*, as well as literature provided by NHS Careers and the Department of Health.

- Find out if your local hospital has open days, and make a particular point of attending.

- Accept any opportunity to undertake caring work in hospital or within the community. This will demonstrate to the colleges that you are serious about a nursing career.

- Gain as much experience as you can of working with people, in a team, in a shop, or by undertaking the Duke of Edinburgh's Award.

What courses and qualifications are available?

To become a registered nurse (RN) or midwife, you must take a pre-registration diploma or a degree course. Get hold of prospectuses to see which courses best suit your interests – not all institutions provide qualifications in all four branches of nursing. Applications are made through the Nursing and Midwives Admissions Service (NMAS) for diploma courses and through the Universities and Colleges Admissions Service (UCAS) for degree courses (see pages 41–42).

Pre-registration courses

The course begins with a Common Foundation Programme (CFP). This enables you to progress into the branch programme by providing you with the knowledge and skills required to care for people in hospital or in the community. This includes, for example: the theory and practice of nursing, sociology, psychology, health education and health. You then follow one of four branch programmes, and normally you must decide at the beginning of your training which of these you wish to choose. They are:

- adult nursing
- mental health nursing
- children's nursing
- learning disability nursing.

During your training you will not be part of the hospital workforce but a student. Time spent in the classroom will be interspersed with periods of work placement. There will be plenty of experience in hospital, residential and community settings. You will watch experienced nurses at work and perform some duties yourself under their supervision. During the later stages you will undertake 1000 hours of rostered service, working as part of the nursing team.

The diploma in higher education is usually three years. Degree courses are three or four years. When researching your courses, remember that course content can vary. You should check which institutions offer the branch programme of most interest to you. Check other details as well – for example, would you have the opportunity to study specialist areas like Clinical Nurse Research, Health Visiting or Cancer Nursing? Would you be interested to move abroad later in your career and therefore would like a course that has a European content and/or language training? All these should be checked with the course providers.

Midwifery courses

There are two ways to qualify as a midwife. The 'direct' route is via a specialist diploma or degree programme in midwifery, without a nursing qualification. If you choose to take a diploma in higher education midwifery course, you may have the opportunity at your college to progress to a top-up year to obtain a BSc Hons Midwifery.

During the first year of diploma and degree courses, you gain insight into midwifery practice and the midwifery profession and also explore general health and illness issues. The second year focuses on both normal and abnormal childbearing, and you will spend more time in the clinical area. During the third year, there is much less theory, and you will begin to function as an independent practitioner while being supported by an experienced midwife.

The second route into midwifery is via a post-registration course – after qualifying as a registered nurse in adult nursing, you can then take a further programme in midwifery.

Accelerated courses

A few institutions offer accelerated nursing courses for graduates who hold a health-related degree. Programmes are modified from existing diploma courses and lead to qualifications in adult nursing, mental health nursing, learning disability nursing or children's nursing. The course lasts a minimum of 24 months.

What about funding?

The tuition fees for both diploma and degree courses are paid by the NHS. Students on a nursing diploma course receive a bursary of at least £4600pa, which is not means tested. Students taking degree courses are entitled to student loans, and may receive a bursary that is means-tested. Contact the NHS Student Grants Unit for information on NHS bursaries, and get hold of the Department of Health leaflet 'Financial Help for Health Students' (see page 42 for addresses).

What publications should I look at?

Careers literature from NHS Careers

- *Nursing and Midwifery in the New NHS: A hundred careers rolled into one*
- *Be Part of the New NHS: Opportunities for qualified healthcare professionals*

Careers advice and education directories

- *Careers in Nursing and Related Professions*, Linda Nazarko, Kogan Page
- *Careers in Social Care,* Bernard Moss, Kogan Page
- *CRAC Degree Course Guides: Medicine & Professions Allied to Medicine;* and *Physiology, Anatomy & Human Biology,* Hobsons Publishing
- *CRAC Directory of Further Education* (DOFE), Hobsons Publishing
- *Degree Course Offers*, Brian Heap, Trotman
- *Getting into Nursing and Midwifery*, Dr Janet Gibbons, Trotman
- *Getting into Paramedical Sciences: A guide to professions allied to medicine,* Joan Llewlyn Owens, Trotman
- *Getting into Physiotherapy,* Trotman
- *Medicine & Allied Profession Courses,* in The Complete Guides series, UCAS/Trotman
- *Nursing: It Makes You Think,* and *Meet Someone New Every Day,* Department of Health

- *Occupations,* COIC
- *The Times A–Z of Careers and Jobs,* Kogan Page
- *University and College Entrance,* UCAS
- *Working in Complementary and Alternative Medicine: A career guide,* Loulou Brown, Kogan Page

Journals

- *Nursing Times*
- *Nursing Standard*
- Check professional bodies as some publish their own journals and newsletters for members.

For more advice on careers and higher education choices, have a look at the resources available through www.careersUK.co.uk

Which addresses will help me?

Advice on nursing careers and training

in England
NHS Careers
PO Box 376
Bristol BS99 3EY
tel: 0845 60 60 655
email: advice@nhscareers.nhs.uk
website: www.nhs.uk/careers

Nurses and Midwives Central Clearing House (NMCCH)
ENB, PO Box 9017
London W1A 0XA
tel: 020 7391 6291/6305/6274/6317

in Northern Ireland
National Board for Nursing, Midwifery and Health Visiting for Northern Ireland
79 Chichester Street, Belfast BT1 4JE
tel: 028 9023 8152
email: enqs@nbni.n-i.nhs.uk

in Scotland
National Board for Nursing, Midwifery and Health Visiting for Scotland
Careers Information Service
22 Queen Street
Edinburgh EH2 1NT
tel: 0131 225 2096
email: careers@nbs.org.uk
website: www.nbs.org.uk

in Wales
**Welsh National Board for Nursing,
Midwifery and Health Visiting**
2nd Floor, Golate House
101 St Mary Street
Cardiff CF1 1DX
tel: 01222 261400
email: info@wnb.org.uk
website: www.wnb.org.uk

Diploma and degree courses

in Scotland (diploma course application package)
NBS Catch
PO Box 21
Edinburgh EH2 1NT
tel: 0131 247 6622
(10am–3pm for application package)

in Northern Ireland
School of Nursing and Midwifery
Registry Office
The Queen's University of Belfast
1–3 College Park East
Belfast BT7 1LQ
tel: 028 9027 3754/028 9033 5116
email: nursing@qub.ac.uk

in England (diploma course application package)
Nursing and Midwives Admissions Service (NMAS)
Rosehill
New Barn Lane
Cheltenham
Gloucestershire GL52 3LZ
tel: 01242 223707
website: www.nmas.ac.uk

in England (degree course application package)
Universities and Colleges Admission Service (UCAS)
Rosehill, New Barn Lane
Cheltenham
Gloucestershire GL52 3LZ
tel: 01242 223707 (or general enquiries: 01242 227788)
website: www.ucas.com

Information on funding

NHS Student Grants Unit
Room 212C, Government Building
Norcross
Blackpool FY5 3TA
tel: 01253 856123

Department of Health
PO Box 777
London SE1 6XH
email: doh@prologistics.co.uk
(leaflet: 'Financial Help for Health Students')

Professional bodies and unions

Community and District Nursing Association
Thames Valley University
Westal House
32–38 Uxbridge Road
London W5 2BS
tel: 020 8280 5032
website: www.cdna.tvu.ac.uk

Institute of Healthcare Management
7–10 Chandos Street
London W1M 9DE
tel: 020 7460 7654
website: www.lhm.org.uk

Royal College of Nursing
RCN Headquarters
20 Cavendish Square
London W1M 0DB
tel: 020 7409 3333
website: www.rcn.org.uk
(Visit the website to find out where your nearest
branch of the RCN is.)

**UKCC (United Kingdom Central Council
for Nursing and Midwifery)**
23 Portland Place
London W1N 4JT
tel: 020 7637 7181
website: www.ukcc.org.uk

UNISON
Mabledon Place
London WC1H 9AJ
tel: 020 7388 2366
website: www.unison.org.uk

More Questions & Answers available from Trotman

Questions & Answers Careers Series

Accountancy
Advertising
Animals
Architecture
Armed Forces
Art & Design, 2nd edition
Banking
Catering & Hotel Management
Child Care
Complementary Medicine
Computing, 2nd edition
Dentistry
Engineering
Environment & Conservation
Fashion & Clothing Design,
  2nd edition
Fire Service
Hairdressing
Journalism
Languages
Law

Library & Information Work
Marketing, 2nd edition
Medicine
Modelling
Music
Nursing, 2nd edition
Office & Secretarial Work
Photography
Physiotherapy
Police
Psychology
Public Relations
Radio, Television & Film,
  2nd edition
Retail, 2nd edition
Science
Social Work
Sport, 2nd edition
Teaching
Theatre, 2nd edition
Tourism, 2nd edition

Questions & Answers Degree Subject Guides

Studying Art & Design
Studying Business &
  Management
Studying Chemical
  Engineering
Studying Computer Science

Studying Drama
Studying English
Studying Law
Studying Media
Studying Psychology
Studying Sports Science